LYME DISEASE DIET PLAN GUIDE BOOK

A Healthy Dietary Plan for Lyme Disease Nutrition and Healthy Eating for Lyme Disease Management

REX LEWIS

Table of Contents

Introduction

Lyme disease Is a Tick-Borne Sickness Caused by the Bacteria Borrelia Burgdorferi. Medical Treatment, Usually Antibiotics, Is The Main Method For Treating Lyme Disease. Some People Also Consider Complementary Techniques, Such As Dietary Changes, To Improve Their General Health. There Is No Special "Lyme Disease Diet" Recommended By Medical Authorities, Therefore Any Dietary Changes Should Be Consulted With A Healthcare Provider.

Advocates Of Alternative And Holistic Methods Propose That Specific Dietary Selections Can Assist In Symptom Management And Boost The Immune

System. The Objectives Of A Lyme Disease Diet, As Suggested By Some, May Involve Minimizing Inflammation, Bolstering The Immune System, And Enhancing Overall Well-Being. Here Are Some Fundamental Guidelines That Patients With Lyme Disease May Want To Include In Their Diet:

• Anti-Inflammatory Foods Can Help Combat Chronic Inflammation Commonly Linked To Lyme Disease. Eating Foods With Anti-Inflammatory Qualities, Like Fatty Fish High In Omega-3 Fatty Acids, Fruits, Vegetables, And Nuts, Can Be Advantageous.

• A Well-Rounded And Nutrient-Dense Diet Is Crucial For Maintaining Overall

Health And Helps Bolster The Immune System. Consuming A Diverse Range Of Fruits, Vegetables, Lean Proteins, And Whole Grains Ensures The Intake Of Vital Vitamins And Minerals.

• Probiotics May Help Alleviate Gastrointestinal Symptoms In Individuals With Lyme Disease. Consuming Probiotic-Rich Foods Such As Yogurt, Kefir, Sauerkraut, And Other Fermented Foods Can Support A Healthy Gut Microbiome.

• Avoiding Trigger Foods: Some People with Lyme disease May Have Sensitivity to Specific Foods. Avoiding Trigger Foods Like Gluten, Dairy, Or Processed Sweets May Help Ease Symptoms.

- **Hydration:** Ensuring Adequate Hydration Is Crucial For Maintaining Good Health And Can Aid The Body's Innate Detoxifying Mechanisms. It Is Advisable To Drink A Sufficient Quantity Of Water.

It Is Essential To Exercise Caution And Seek Guidance From A Healthcare Expert, Such As A Qualified Dietitian Or Physician, Particularly When Dealing With A Complicated Condition Like Lyme Disease. Moreover, Individual Reactions To Dietary Modifications Can Differ, And What Is Effective For One Individual May Not Be Effective For Another. Medical Treatment Is The Major Evidence-Based Method For Managing Lyme

Disease, And Any Changes In Diet Should Support But Not Substitute Recommended Medical Treatments.

CHAPTER ONE
What Is Lyme disease?

Lyme disease Is an Infection Caused by the Spirochete Bacterium Borrelia Burgdorferi. The Main Mode Of Transmission To Humans Is By The Biting Of Infected Black-Legged Ticks, Often Known As Deer Ticks (Ixodes Scapularis Or Ixodes Pacificus). Ticks Are Common in Wooded and Grassy Regions and Can Transmit Germs through Their Bite, Potentially Causing Lyme disease.

Common Signs of Lyme disease Are:

• Erythema Migrans (EM) Rash Is Frequently One Of The Initial And Most Identifiable Indications Of Lyme Disease. The Typical Presentation Of

Lyme disease Is A Circular, Red Rash With A Bull's-Eye Pattern Around The Tick Bite Location, Although Not All Individuals With Lyme Disease Will Exhibit This Rash.

• Symptoms Resembling Those Of Influenza: Common Symptoms In The Early Stages Of The Disease Include Fever, Chills, Lethargy, Headache, Muscle, And Joint Aches.

• Neurological Symptoms of Lyme disease May Include Numbness, Tingling, Bell's palsy, And Cognitive Impairment.

• Lyme Illness Can Result In Joint Inflammation, Causing Symptoms

Similar To Arthritis, Especially In The Knees.

Untreated Lyme disease Can Advance to More Severe and Enduring Symptoms, Impacting Different Organs and Systems in the Body. Prompt Diagnosis And Treatment With Antibiotics Are Essential For Effectively Controlling The Illness And Avoiding Consequences.

Not All Tick Bites Lead To Lyme disease. The Transmission Of The Bacterium Usually Occurs When The Tick Is Attached For A Prolonged Duration, Often 24 To 48 Hours. Utilizing Prevention Strategies Including Insect Repellent, Protective Clothes, And Thorough Tick Checks

Post Outside Activities Will Lower The Chances Of Getting Lyme Disease. If Someone Feels They Have Been Bitten By A Tick Carrying An Infection Or Has Symptoms Typical Of Lyme Disease, They Should Promptly Seek Medical Assistance For Accurate Diagnosis And Treatment.

Causes and Symptoms

Causes: Lyme disease Is Primarily Caused by the Bacteria Borrelia Burgdorferi, Which Is Spread To Humans Through The Bite Of Infected Black-Legged Ticks (Ixodes Scapularis Or Ixodes Pacificus). Ticks Acquire The Bacteria Through Eating On Infected Animals Like Mice And Deer. Not All Ticks Are Carriers Of The Bacteria,

And Transmission Normally Happens After The Tick Has Been Attached For A Prolonged Period, Often 24 To 48 Hours.

Lyme disease Is Not Spread Directly between People; It Is Contracted by the Bite of a Tick Carrying the Virus.

Lyme disease Symptoms Can Vary and Typically Manifest in Stages. Symptoms Might Vary In Severity And Progression From Person To Person. Typical Symptoms Include:

1. **Erythema Migrans (EM) Rash**: A Circular, Red Rash With A Bull's-Eye Pattern That Develops At The Location Of The Tick Bite. Nevertheless, Not All

Individuals With Lyme Disease Have This Rash.

2. Symptoms Like Those Of The Flu, Such As Fever, Chills, Weariness, Headache, And Muscle And Joint Aches, Are Frequently Observed In The Initial Phases Of The Illness.

3. Lyme disease can Impact the Nerve System, Causing Symptoms Like Numbness, Tingling, Bell's Palsy, And Cognitive Difficulties.

4. Joint Discomfort Can Occur Due To Inflammation In The Joints, Especially In The Knees, Leading To Sensations Similar To Arthritis.

5. In Rare Instances, Lyme disease Can Impact The Heart, Leading To

Symptoms Including Chest Discomfort And Irregular Heartbeats.

6. Ocular Inflammation: Some People May Develop Inflammation In The Eyes, Resulting In Redness And Light Sensitivity.

Delayed Diagnosis And Treatment Of Lyme Disease Can Lead To The Emergence Of More Severe And Chronic Symptoms That Impact Multiple Organs And Systems In The Body. These May Involve Persistent Joint Inflammation, Neurological Problems, And Heart-Related Difficulties.

It Is Essential To Promptly Seek Medical Care If Someone Feels They

Have Been Bitten By An Infected Tick Or If They Exhibit Symptoms Indicative Of Lyme Disease. Timely Identification And Suitable Antibiotic Therapy Are Crucial In Halting The Advancement Of The Infection And Reducing Potential Consequences.

CHAPTER TWO
Diagnosis and Treatment Options

Diagnosis: Diagnosing Lyme Disease Requires A Comprehensive Assessment That Includes Clinical Evaluation, Medical History, And Laboratory Investigations. The Essential Elements Of The Diagnostic Process Are:

• Healthcare Practitioners Will Do A Clinical Evaluation By Assessing The Patient's Symptoms, Medical History, And Potential Exposure To Tick Habitats. The Appearance Of The Erythema Migrans (EM) Rash Is Frequently A Significant Signal.

• Laboratory Testing Are Utilized To Confirm A Diagnosis When The

Normal Rash Is Not Present Or The Symptoms Are Unusual, Notwithstanding The Need Of Clinical Evaluation. There Are Two Main Categories Of Laboratory Tests:

• Enzyme-Linked Immunosorbent Assay (ELISA) Is Commonly Used As The First Step In Blood Testing. A Confirmatory Test Is Conducted If The ELISA Result Is Positive Or Inconclusive.

• A Western Blot Test Is Used To Confirm The Diagnosis Of Lyme Disease By Identifying Particular Antibodies To The Bacteria That Causes The Disease.

• **Treatment:** The Main Approach For Lyme Disease Is Antibiotics, And Prompt Action Is Crucial To Stop The Infection From Advancing And Problems From Arising. Some Frequently Prescribed Antibiotics Are:

Doxycycline Is A Commonly Prescribed Antibiotic For Individuals Aged 8 And Above.

• Amoxicillin Or Cefuroxime Are Frequently Used For Pregnant Women, Nursing Mothers, And Young Children.

• The Duration Of Antibiotic Therapy Fluctuates Based On The Disease's Stage And Symptom Severity. Typically, A Two To Four-Week

Regimen Of Antibiotics Is Adequate For Treating Early-Stage Lyme Disease.

• For Patients Experiencing Chronic Symptoms Or Problems, Additional Or Extended Rounds Of Antibiotics May Be Required. The Use Of Extended Antibiotics Is A Topic Of Controversy In The Medical Field, And Treatment Length Decisions Should Be Decided In Collaboration With A Healthcare Provider.

Self-Diagnosis And Self-Treatment For Lyme disease Are Not Recommended. It Is Essential To Promptly Seek Medical Attention If There Is Suspicion Of Exposure To Infected Ticks Or The Presence Of Symptoms For Correct

Diagnosis And Suitable Treatment. Preventive Actions, Such Preventing Tick Bites And Rapidly Removing Ticks, Are Crucial For Minimizing The Risk Of Lyme Disease.

The Impact of Diet on Lyme disease Symptoms

Diet May Help Manage Symptoms Of Lyme Disease For Some People, But It Should Be Used In Addition To, Not Instead Of, Traditional Medical Care. Individuals With Lyme Disease May Exhibit A Variety Of Symptoms And Have Diverse Reactions To Various Meals. Here Are Several Ways In Which Nutrition Might Impact Lyme Disease Symptoms:

1. Lyme Illness Can Induce Inflammation In The Body. Some Diets, Such Those Containing Refined Sugars, Processed Ingredients, And Bad Fats, Can Lead To Inflammation. An Anti-Inflammatory Diet Containing Fruits, Vegetables, Omega-3 Fatty Acids, And Antioxidants Can Reduce Inflammation.

2. Gut Health: Certain Patients With Lyme disease May Encounter Gastrointestinal Problems. Consuming Probiotic-Rich Foods Like Yogurt, Kefir, Sauerkraut, And Other Fermented Foods Help Promote A Healthy Gut Microbiome. Ensuring Optimal Gut Health Is Crucial For

General Well-Being And Immune System Efficiency.

3. Food Sensitivity: Individuals With Lyme Disease May Experience Sensitivity To Specific Foods. Typical Triggers Include Of Gluten, Dairy, And Processed Sweets. It Can Be Helpful To Identify And Avoid Certain Meals That May Worsen Symptoms. This Method May Require Following An Elimination Diet Or Consulting With A Healthcare Practitioner.

4. Nutrient Density: Lyme Disease Can Affect The Absorption And Use Of Nutrients. Consuming A Nutrient-Rich Diet Consisting Of A Diverse Range Of Fruits, Vegetables, Lean Proteins, And Whole Grains Is Crucial For Obtaining

Critical Vitamins And Minerals That Promote General Health And Boost The Immune System.

5. Adequate Hydration Is Essential For Facilitating The Body's Innate Detoxifying Mechanisms. Sufficient Water Consumption Aids In Eliminating Toxins From The Body And Enhances General Well-Being.

It Is Crucial To Carefully Consider Dietary Modifications And Tailor Advice To Fit An Individual's Unique Requirements And Tolerances. Seeking Guidance From A Healthcare Expert, Namely A Registered Dietitian Or Nutritionist, Can Assist In Developing A Customized Nutrition Plan Based On The Individual's Health

Condition, Symptoms, And Dietary Choices.

Diet Can Enhance General Health, But It Should Not Be Used As A Replacement For Medical Care. Timely And Suitable Medical Treatment For Lyme Disease Usually Includes Antibiotics Given By A Healthcare Provider. Consult A Healthcare Provider Before Making Any Dietary Changes To Verify They Are In Line With The Individual's Treatment Plan And Medical Requirements.

Building a Foundation: Essential Nutrients for Lyme disease Recovery

Establishing A Base For Recovering From Lyme Disease Entails Prioritizing A Diet High In Nutrients To Promote General Health And Strengthen The Immune System. Although Individual Requirements May Differ, The Basic Nutrients Listed Below Can Aid In Promoting Recovery:

• Antioxidants Combat Oxidative Stress and Inflammation. Include A Diverse Selection Of Vibrant Fruits And Vegetables Including Berries, Citrus Fruits, Leafy Greens, And Bell Peppers, As They Are Abundant In

Vitamins C And E, Beta-Carotene, And Other Antioxidants.

- Omega-3 Fatty Acids, Present In Fatty Fish Like Salmon, Mackerel, And Sardines, As Well As In Flaxseeds, Chia Seeds, And Walnuts, Possess Anti-Inflammatory Qualities And Can Promote Joint Health And General Well-Being.

- Adequate Protein Is Crucial For Tissue Repair And Immunological Function. Incorporate Low-Fat Protein Sources Like Poultry, Fish, Legumes, Tofu, And Nuts Into Your Diet.

Nutrients: Vitamins and Minerals

- Vitamin D Is Crucial For Immunological Function And Bone

Health. Sources Of Vitamin D Include Sunlight, Fatty Fish, Fortified Dairy Or Plant-Based Milk, And Supplements If Necessary.

• B Vitamins Aid in Energy Metabolism And Nervous System Function. Incorporate Whole Grains, Leafy Greens, Legumes, And Lean Meats.

• Zinc Is Crucial For Immunological Function And Wound Healing. Lean Meats, Dairy, Nuts, And Seeds Are Nutritious Sources Of Food.

• Probiotics Are Beneficial For Gut Health, Which Is Important Because Lyme Illness Can Impact The Digestive System. Incorporate Fermented Foods

Such As Yogurt, Kefir, Sauerkraut, And Kimchi.

• Adequate Hydration Is Crucial For Detoxing And Maintaining Overall Health. Stay Hydrated By Consuming A Sufficient Quantity Of Water During The Day.

• Fiber, Present In Fruits, Vegetables, Whole Grains, And Legumes, Promotes Digestive Health And Aids In Managing Gastrointestinal Symptoms.

• Iron Is Crucial For Preventing Anemia And Maintaining Energy Levels. Excellent Sources Consist Of Lean Meats, Chicken, Fish, Beans, Lentils, And Fortified Cereals.

• Magnesium Aids In Muscle And Nerve Function And May Improve Sleep Quality. Sources Consist Of Leafy Greens, Nuts, Seeds, Whole Grains, And Legumes.

• Caloric Adequacy: Make Sure You Are Ingesting A Sufficient Amount Of Calories To Meet Your Energy Requirements And Aid In Recuperation. This Is Crucial, Particularly If Lyme Illness Has Impacted Your Appetite.

It Is Essential To Customize Dietary Selections Based On Individual Tastes And Sensitivities. Seeking Advice From A Healthcare Professional, Such A Registered Dietitian, Can Offer Individualized Recommendations.

Individual Responses To Specific Meals Can Vary, Therefore It Is Advantageous To Observe How Your Body Reacts To Different Nutrients And Modify Your Diet Accordingly. A Balanced Diet, Along With Medical Treatment Provided By A Healthcare Expert, Is A Comprehensive Strategy To Recovering From Lyme Disease.

CHAPTER THREE
The Lyme disease Diet Plan

Although There Is No Officially Recommended "Lyme Disease Diet" By The Medical Profession, Some People With Lyme Disease Consider Making Dietary Adjustments To Improve Their General Health And Alleviate Symptoms. It Is Crucial To Consult A Healthcare Practitioner Before Making Any Dietary Changes To Receive Specific Counsel Tailored To Particular Health Conditions, Requirements, And Sensitivities. Here Is A Basic Outline For A Possible Diet Plan For Lyme disease.

1. Focus On Anti-Inflammatory Foods:

• Include A Variety Of Fruits And Vegetables Rich In Antioxidants, Such As Berries, Citrus Fruits, Leafy Greens, And Colorful Vegetables.

• Choose Fatty Fish High In Omega-3 Fatty Acids, Such As Salmon, Mackerel, And Sardines.

• Incorporate Nuts and Seeds, Like Flaxseeds And Walnuts, Which Also Provide Omega-3s.

2. Lean Protein Sources:

• Include Lean Protein To Support Muscle Repair And Immune Function. Options Include Poultry, Fish, Tofu, Legumes, And Beans.

3. Whole Grains:

• Choose Whole Grains Like Brown Rice, Quinoa, Oats, And Whole Wheat To Provide Fiber, Vitamins, And Minerals.

4. Probiotic-Rich Foods:

• Support Gut Health With Probiotics Found In Fermented Foods Like Yogurt, Kefir, Sauerkraut, Kimchi, And Pickles.

5. Hydration:

• Stay Well-Hydrated With Water, Herbal Teas, And Broths To Support Detoxification And Overall Health.

6. Foods Rich In Vitamins And Minerals:

• Ensure A Well-Rounded Intake Of Vitamins And Minerals By Incorporating A Variety Of Foods:

• **Vitamin C:** Citrus Fruits, Strawberries, Bell Peppers.

• **Vitamin D:** Fatty Fish, Fortified Dairy Or Plant-Based Milk, Exposure To Sunlight.

• **B Vitamins:** Whole Grains, Leafy Greens, Lean Proteins.

• **Zinc:** Lean Meats, Dairy, Nuts, Seeds.

• **Iron:** Lean Meats, Poultry, Fish, Beans, Lentils, Fortified Cereals.

- **Magnesium:** Leafy Greens, Nuts, Seeds, Whole Grains, Legumes.

7. Avoid Potential Trigger Foods:

• Identify And Avoid Foods That May Trigger Symptoms. Common Triggers Include Gluten, Dairy, And Processed Sugars. An Elimination Diet May Help Identify Sensitivities.

8. Caloric Adequacy:

• Ensure You Are Consuming Enough Calories To Support Energy Needs And Recovery. Adjust Portion Sizes Based On Individual Activity Levels And Metabolic Needs.

9. Personalized Approach:

• Consider Individual Preferences And Sensitivities When Creating A Dietary Plan. Consult With A Healthcare Professional, Such As A Registered Dietitian, For Personalized Guidance.

It Is Important To Follow A Well-Rounded And Diverse Diet That Offers Necessary Nutrients, Promotes General Well-Being, And Is Customized To Personal Requirements. Furthermore, It Is Important To Consult Healthcare Specialists About Dietary Modifications To Ensure They Are Consistent With The Comprehensive Treatment Regimen For Lyme Disease. Individual Reactions To Meals Can

Differ, So It's Crucial To Observe How Your Body Responds And Modify Your Diet Accordingly.

Stress Management Techniques

Effective Stress Management Is Essential For Maintaining General Well-Being, Particularly In Times Of Adversity, Such As When Facing Health Conditions Like Lyme Disease. Here Are Few Stress Management Practices That May Be Beneficial:

• Engage In Deep Breathing Exercises To Stimulate The Body's Relaxation Response. Breathe In Deeply Through Your Nostrils, Pause Briefly, Then Breathe Out Slowly Through Your Mouth.

• Practice Mindfulness Meditation To Focus Your Attention On The Present Moment. Concentrate On Your Breath, Feelings, Or A Specific Focal Point, Letting Thoughts Pass Without Judgment.

• Engage In Progressive Muscle Relaxation (PMR) By Deliberately Tensing And Then Relaxing Various Muscle Groups In Your Body. This Aids In Promoting Bodily Relaxation And Can Decrease Overall Tension.

• Yoga Involves A Combination Of Physical Postures, Breath Control, And Meditation. It Enhances Flexibility, Decreases Muscle Tension, And Fosters A Feeling Of Tranquility.

• Utilize Guided Imagery Or Visualization To Construct A Mental Representation Of A Tranquil And Soothing Environment. This Can Assist In Redirecting Your Attention From Sources Of Stress.

• Engage In Consistent Physical Activity To Release Endorphins, Which Are Natural Mood Enhancers. Select Activities That You Find Enjoyable, Like Walking, Jogging, Swimming, Or Dancing.

• Journaling Involves Recording Your Thoughts And Emotions In A Journal. This Can Aid In Achieving Clarity, Articulating Emotions, And Pinpointing Stressors. Considering The

Favorable Aspects Of Your Life Might Also Be Advantageous.

• Utilize Social Support By Engaging With Friends, Family, Or A Support Group. Expressing Your Emotions And Sharing Your Experiences With Others Can Offer Emotional Assistance And Foster A Feeling Of Belonging To A Group.

• Efficiently Manage Your Time By Organizing It Effectively. Divide Activities Into Smaller, More Manageable Segments, Prioritize Them, And Establish Achievable Objectives. This Can Aid In Decreasing Feelings Of Overwhelm.

• Avoid Consuming Stimulants Such As Caffeine, Particularly In The Evening, As They Can Increase Stress Levels And Interfere With Sleep.

• Adequate Rest: Make Sure You Are Obtaining Sufficient High-Quality Sleep. Develop A Consistent Sleep Schedule And Set Up A Cozy Sleeping Space.

• **Hobbies And Relaxation Activities:** Participate In Activities That You Find Enjoyable, Such As Reading, Listening To Music, Gardening, Or Any Other Pastime That Provides You Happiness And Relaxation.

• **Professional Support:** Consider Consulting A Mental Health

Professional, Like A Therapist Or Counselor, To Discuss Coping Skills And Receive Further Help.

It Is Crucial To Explore Many Ways To Choose The Most Effective Approach For You. Integrating Several Tactics Into Your Daily Routine Can Help Effectively Manage Stress. If Stress Becomes Too Much, Get Professional Help To Create A Personalized Strategy For Handling Stress And Preserving Mental Health.

CHAPTER FOUR
Herbal Supplements

Certain Lyme disease Patients May Benefit from the Inclusion of Herbal Supplements, Which Are Composed Of Plant-Based Substances And Plant Extracts, In Their Dietary Regimen. It Is Imperative To Exercise Prudence When Considering Herbal Supplements And To Seek Guidance From A Healthcare Professional Due To The Potential For Drug Interactions And Individual Incompatibility. The Subsequent Herbal Supplements Have Been The Subject Of Scientific Investigation Or Have Been Utilized By Individuals With Lyme Disease:

1. Cat's Claw (Uncaria Tomentosa):
Some Consider Cat's Claw To Possess Anti-Inflammatory And Immune-Boosting Properties. However, Limited Evidence Supports Its Efficacy In The Treatment Of Lyme Disease, And It May Interact Negatively With Certain Medications.

2. Japanese Knotweed (Polygonum Cuspidatum): Resveratrol And Anti-Inflammatory Properties Are Abundant In Japanese Knotweed. Although Some Individuals Incorporate It Into Their Strategy For Managing The Symptoms Of Lyme Disease, Additional Research Is Required To Ascertain Its Efficacy.

3. Andrographis, Scientifically Known As Andrographis Paniculata, Is A Herb That Possesses Anti-Inflammatory And Immune-Modulating Properties. Although Some People Claim To Use It To Boost Their Immune Systems, Scientific Evidence Is Limited.

4. Samento, A Specific Chemotype Of Cat's Claw Composed Of Pentacyclic Alkaloid, Is Utilized By Certain Individuals Under The Guise That It Possesses More Potent Immune-Modulating Properties. However, There Is A Dearth Of Scientific Evidence.

5. Garlic (Allium Sativum): Garlic Possesses Immune-Boosting And Antimicrobial Properties. Although It

Potentially Benefits Overall Health, Its Precise Effectiveness In The Treatment Of Lyme Disease Remains Uncertain.

6. Resveratrol, An Antioxidant Compound Present In Japanese Knotweed And Red Grapes, Exhibits Promise As An Anti-Inflammatory Agent. It Is Utilized By Some For Its Alleged Health Benefits.

7. Curcumin, the Bioactive Constituent of Turmeric (Curcuma Longa), Exhibits Anti-Inflammatory Characteristics. Although It Potentially Offers Advantages For General Well-Being, The Precise Effects It Has On Lyme Disease Remain Uncertain.

It Is Imperative To Underscore That Herbal Supplements Ought Not To Serve As A Substitute For Medical Treatment Of Lyme Disease, Which Customarily Entails The Administration Of Antibiotics As Prescribed By Medical Practitioners. In Addition, Herbal Supplements May Interact With Medications, Cause Adverse Effects, And Differ In Quality; Therefore, Prior To Incorporating Them Into Your Regimen, It Is Imperative That You Consult A Healthcare Professional.

Consult A Knowledgeable Healthcare Professional, Such As A Naturopathic Doctor Or Integrative Medicine Practitioner, Before Deciding To Take

Herbal Supplements. Such A Professional Can Offer Guidance Tailored To Your Specific Health Condition And Requirements. To Ensure Coordinated And Safe Care, It Is Imperative That You Consistently Communicate Any Supplements You Are Taking To Your Healthcare Team.

Navigating Challenges and Staying Motivated

Managing Lyme Disease Can Be Physically And Emotionally Difficult, Requiring Perseverance And Motivation To Overcome Challenges. Here Are Some Techniques To Assist You In Overcoming Obstacles And Sustaining Motivation:

1. Acquire Knowledge: Familiarize Yourself With Lyme Disease, Its Symptoms, And Treatment Options. Comprehending Your Situation Can Give You The Ability To Make Knowledgeable Choices Regarding Your Health.

2. Establish A Support System By Surrounding Oneself With A Network Of Supportive Friends, Family, And Healthcare Professionals. Confide In Trusted Others About Your Experiences, Emotions, And Worries.

3. Establish Achievable Objectives By Dividing Complex Tasks Into Smaller, More Attainable Goals. Recognize And Celebrate Minor Accomplishments As You Make Progress.

4. Be Attentive To Your Body's Cues And Adapt Your Activity Accordingly. Take Breaks When Necessary And Avoid Overexertion.

5. Prioritize Self-Care By Engaging In Activities That Enhance Physical And Emotional Well-Being, Such As Maintaining A Balanced Diet, Getting Enough Sleep, And Managing Stress.

6. Utilize Mind-Body Approaches Like Mindfulness, Meditation, Or Yoga To Effectively Handle Stress And Enhance Overall Resilience.

7. Seek Assistance From Mental Health Providers Specializing In Chronic Illness Or With Expertise In Lyme Disease.

Acknowledge And Celebrate Your Accomplishments, Even The Minor Ones. Positive Reinforcement Can Enhance Motivation.

9. Manage Your Expectations By Being Realistic About Your Daily Goals. Manage Your Expectations And Practice Self-Compassion During Difficult Periods.

10. Maintain Connections With Your Social Groups, Even If It's Through Virtual Methods. Emotional Well-Being Is Highly Dependent On Social Assistance.

11. Engage In Activities That Bring You Pleasure And A Feeling Of Achievement. Discover Activities That

Resonate With You, Whether They Are Hobbies, Spending Time In Nature, Or Indulging In Creative Efforts.

12. Demonstrate Flexibility And Adaptability By Being Open To Adjustments In Your Treatment Plan Or Daily Routine. Adaptations Could Be Required, And A Versatile Attitude Might Minimize Irritation.

13. Concentrate On Areas Within Your Control, Like Lifestyle Choices, Self-Care Habits, And Mentality.

14. Maintain A Good Mindset By Concentrating On The Elements In Your Life That Generate Happiness And Appreciation. Having A Good Mindset Can Enhance Resilience.

Celebrate Progress Rather Than Perfection By Acknowledging That Advancements May Occur Gradually. Embrace The Process And Acknowledge Your Hard Work Instead Of Striving For Flawlessness.

Managing A Chronic Condition Such As Lyme Disease Is A Process, And It Is OK To Seek Assistance When Necessary. It Is Crucial To Have Open Communication With Your Healthcare Provider And Modify Your Self-Care Practice As Needed. Commend Your Ability To Bounce Back And Acknowledge The Advancements You Achieve As You Move Forward.

Conclusion

Ultimately, Managing Lyme Disease Necessitates A Thorough And Personalized Strategy That Includes Medical Care, Lifestyle Modifications, And Mental Health. It Is Necessary To Comprehend The Causes, Symptoms, And Therapies Available. Seeking Competent Medical Counsel Is Crucial For An Accurate Diagnosis And Treatment Plan.

• Aside From Medical Treatments, Maintaining A Balanced And Nutrient-Dense Diet, Utilizing Stress Management Strategies, And Embracing A Positive Outlook Can Enhance One's Overall Well-Being. It Is Crucial To Be Cautious While Making

Dietary Adjustments And Using Herbal Supplements, And It Is Advisable To Consult Healthcare Professionals To Verify They Are In Line With Your Treatment Plan.

• Establishing A Support Network, Creating Achievable Objectives, And Giving Importance To Self-Care Are Crucial Elements In Handling Lyme Illness. Recognizing And Appreciating Little Achievements, Keeping Social Connections, And Participating In Enjoyable Activities Can Help Sustain Motivation In Difficult Circumstances.

• Each Person's Encounter With Lyme Disease Is Distinct, And There Is No Universal Solution. Collaborate With Your Healthcare Team, Which Includes

Medical Specialists And Mental Health Experts, To Create A Customized Plan That Addresses Your Individual Requirements And Enhances Your Overall Health.

As You Face The Difficulties Of Lyme Illness, Practice Patience, Seek Assistance When Necessary, And Concentrate On The Path Of Improvement And Strength. By Adopting A Thorough And All-Encompassing Strategy, You May Improve Your Quality Of Life And Effectively Address Lyme Disease.

THE END